Oliver Jordan

Nutrition - Everything You Need to Know

Date of Publication - 2018

Trademarks

Liability

Part One - Nutrition

What is it?

Nutrition is the name given to the process by which
all living creatures absorb compounds essential for life.
These compounds are known as nutrients and include
fats, carbohydrates, proteins, minerals, vitamins and
water. With them, we can generate the energy we
need to function, regulate and repair ourselves.

However, for optimum health, our bodies need other
things as well, one of the most important of which is
fibre. This is found only in plants - meat and fish do
not contain any.

Fibre is an essential part of a healthy, balanced diet
and helps prevent heart disease, diabetes, weight gain
and some cancers. It also improves digestive health.
Another is calcium - this is a compound used to build
and maintain bones

However, a nutritious diet is just one factor in
achieving good health. It's also important that the
energy created by nutrition, i.e. calories, is put to good
use. If it isn't, two things happen:

The first is that the body stores the energy as fat in
the

anticipation that it may be needed at some other time - essentially, it's a backup. Exactly the same thing happens if you eat too much - the body has more energy than it can use and rather than just throw it away, it stores it in the form of fat for a rainy day.

Secondly, our bodies are controlled by muscles, and without them we can do absolutely nothing. The more we use these muscles, the stronger and more efficient they become. This leads to increased physical strength, endurance and stamina. Our organs are controlled by muscles as well. For example, cardiac muscle in the heart is responsible for pumping blood around the body. The stronger all these muscles are, the greater the overall health of the body.

However, if we don't exercise to use the energy, the opposite happens. Our muscles become weak and so we are able to do less physically - everything becomes an effort. More dangerous, however, is the effect on our vital organs, such as the heart, lungs, liver and the kidneys. Weak, under-used muscles in any of these results in reduced functionality that make us feel unwell, restrict our ability to do basic things and, ultimately, are the cause of illness, disease and, all too often, premature death.

Our diets can also be affected by factors such as genetics, our environment, age and culture. Many people have to take these into account when deciding what they can and cannot eat. For example, there may be a family history of heart disease, or risk factors such as high blood pressure, that rule certain foods out. Young and active people need more food than older or less active ones. Also, people who are trying to lose weight can find it difficult to get the nutrients they need due to their necessarily restricted diet.

In this book, I show how to ensure you have a healthy, balanced diet that will keep your body firing on all cylinders. This will, without doubt, be the single most effective thing you can do, to not just feel good but also vastly reduce the likelihood of getting dangerous conditions and diseases.

The ones I am talking about are cancer, heart disease, stroke, high blood pressure, diabetes and osteoporosis. Currently, these are all rife, particularly in the western hemisphere, and ruin millions of lives every year. Much of it is preventable and a healthy diet is the starting point.

Some pertinent quotes:

"Let food be your medicine, and medicine be your food" - Hippocrates

"He who has health has hope, and he who has hope has everything." - Arabian Proverb

Nutritional Status

Nutritional status is basically an assessment of a person's body from a dietary standpoint. Factors taken into account are what the person eats, the types of nutrient in their body, and if there are enough of those nutrients to enable them to function efficiently.

More specifically, the assessment looks at the essential nutrients. These come in two classes:

1) Macronutrients - these are nutrients that generate the large amount of energy the body needs in order to grow and maintain itself. They are found in fats, protein and carbohydrates

2) Micronutrients - found in vitamins and minerals, these play a vital role in the body's general health and well-being

Other factors considered include appearance and the blood levels of various compounds. How a person looks will give a dietician a lot of information. For example, the condition of their skin, hair and nails offers clear clues as to how well nourished they are.

The presence of normal amounts of fat and muscle does as well. The dietician can also check that the person's weight is appropriate for their height, i.e. their body mass index (BMI).

A blood test is a more scientific method of assessing someone's nutritional status. It does this by showing what's in their blood and so, by extension, what's in their body. For example, a person who is malnourished will have low levels of certain proteins. A high level of cholesterol indicates a person may drink too much alcohol. A blood test can also highlight irregularities in body functions that need to be treated with an appropriate diet.

Factors such as access to food, existing chronic conditions, and the ability to eat food, are also indicators of nutritional status. As are certain medical conditions, such as Crohn's disease, that limit a person's ability to absorb nutrients from food they've eaten.

Sadly, despite the clear benefits of having their nutritional status assessed, very few people ever think to have it done. Indeed, many people have never even heard of it. In most cases, it's the fact they are putting on excess weight that eventually persuades them something is amiss.

However, if something is wrong internally, it won't be so obvious. For this reason, I suggest everyone should have their nutritional status checked periodically. Many people are shaken by the results.

Recognising Nutrient Deficiencies

It is a known fact that the vast majority of people have a diet that does not provide all the nutrients required for a long and healthy life. Given that in most parts of the world there is no shortage of food, this does seem perverse.

One reason for it is ignorance - many people just don't realise how important a balanced diet actually is. Other reasons are stupidity, laziness and lack of self-control. Many people are simply too idle, or too silly, to cook proper food. Instead, they rely on fried chicken and fish, pizzas, and other types of processed food. Indeed, many people are quite happy to eat food that they know isn't good for them.

Even people who are aware of the importance of their diet, and take care to ensure they are eating healthily, still get caught out. One way this can happen is that they get a condition that affects their ability to absorb nutrients. Another common cause is the big processed food corporations. All too often, they sell us food that is not as rich in a particular nutrient as they would have us believe.

Luckily, most nutrient deficiencies eventually manifest themselves in one way or another - some you can see, some you can feel and some you can hear. The trick is spotting the signs, being able to interpret them and acting on them.

Lets take a look at the most common nutrient deficiencies:

Iron
About a quarter of the world's population is thought to be deficient in iron. This essential mineral is found in every cell in the body, and is used to make oxygen-carrying proteins called haemoglobin and myoglobin.

When your iron level is too low, you become anaemic. This is a condition whereby the lack of iron in the body causes a reduction in the number of red blood cells. As these store and carry oxygen in the blood, having less of them than you should means your organs and tissues won't get as much oxygen as they need.

The most common symptoms are tiredness and lethargy, shortness of breath and heart palpitations. You may also experience headaches, tinnitus, loss of hair, impaired sense of taste and difficulty swallowing. Furthermore, it can make you more susceptible to illness and infection, as it adversely affects your immune system.

Iron deficiency is not necessarily diet related. It can

also be caused by stomach ulcers, stomach and bowel cancer, and by taking non-steroidal anti-inflammatory drugs.

Good sources of iron include fish, eggs, leafy green vegetables, brown rice, beans, nuts, seeds, meat and dried fruit.

Iodine

A large proportion of the world's population is affected by iodine deficiency. This is a mineral that is essential for the production of thyroid hormones. These ensure the body's metabolic rate – the speed at which chemical reactions take place – are optimal.

The most common symptom is a swelling of the thyroid gland, which causes a lump to form in the front of the neck. Others include a dry mouth, dry skin, poor memory and concentration, an increase in heart rate and shortness of breath. Severe cases (with children in particular) can cause mental retardation and abnormal development.

One of the best ways to get iodine is to eat sea vegetables, such as kelp, nori, kombu and wakame. Other good sources are eggs, fish and dairy produce. You can also get small amounts of iodine from fruit and vegetables - this is largely dependent though on factors such as soil quality, the type of fertilizer used and the method of irrigation.

Vitamin D

Vitamin D is a fat-soluble vitamin that helps to regulate the amounts of calcium and phosphate in our bodies. These nutrients are required to keep our bones, teeth and muscles healthy. Deficiencies can cause bone deformities, such as rickets in children, and a condition called osteomalacia (bone ache) in adults.

Symptoms that indicate a lack of vitamin D are depression, excessive head sweating, fatigue and general aches and pains. A deficiency in vitamin D is not usually obvious, however, as it often develops gradually, and thus unnoticed, over a period of time.

Unlike most vitamins that can only be acquired from the foods we eat, vitamin D is made by the body. So although some foods do contain small quantities of it, diet isn't really a factor. What *is* important is sunlight. Our bodies manufacture vitamin D from cholesterol in the skin when it is exposed to the sun. And, as many people don't get enough exposure to the sun, they don't have enough vitamin D.

This is the best way to get it - fifteen minutes of sun twice a week is enough for most people. Foods such as oily fish, red meat, liver and eggs are the best dietary sources, albeit a poor second best. It is also possible to get vitamin D in the form of pill supplements.

Calcium

Calcium is a mineral that's essential for life. In addition to building teeth and bones, and maintaining them, it helps our blood clot, enables our nerves to send messages around the body, and helps our muscles to contract and expand.

A diet deficient in calcium does not produce obvious symptoms in the short-term because the body maintains its calcium level by taking it from bone when supplies are low. Over the long-term, however, this weakens the bones and can result in osteoporosis and, with children, rickets. Both increase the likelihood of bone fractures.

A good source of calcium is unboned fish - one tin of sardines provides nearly 50 percent of the recommended daily amount. Others include dairy products and dark green leafy vegetables. Some people take calcium supplements but this really isn't necessary given that it's present in so many foods.

Magnesium

Magnesium is crucial to nerve transmission, muscle contraction, blood coagulation, energy production, nutrient metabolism, and bone and cell formation.

Nearly 50 percent of people are lacking in this essential nutrient.

As it plays such an important role in so many of the body's functions, a magnesium deficiency can have a large number of symptoms. These include difficulty sleeping, facial tics, cramps, eye twitching, migraines, loss of appetite, headaches and nausea. It can also be the cause of numbness, seizures, abnormal heart rhythms and personality changes.

The best source of magnesium is almonds - a handful of these nuts provides around fifteen percent of the recommended daily amount. Cashews and peanuts are not far behind. Also good are avocados, beans (black in particular), grains, potatoes, brown rice, yoghurt and leafy green vegetables, spinach especially.

You should also be aware that certain foods and drinks can deplete the level of magnesium in your body. Regular consumption of foods high in sugar - cakes, candy, biscuits, pastries, etc - causes the body to excrete magnesium via the kidneys.

Ditto caffeinated drinks like tea and coffee, carbonated drinks like soda, and also alcohol. Certain drugs, including diuretics, heart and asthma medication, and birth control pills do the same.

Nutrition Myths

Nutrition research has come a long way in the last few years. Despite this, however, a lot of people still give credence to outdated theories and ideas. For example, that fat is bad for you, eating eggs raises cholesterol and that gluten should be avoided Many of these have come about due to simple misconceptions. Others are due to a deliberate policy of misinformation by food manufacturers. Then there's the Internet - the first port of call for many people when they decide to alter their diet. Unfortunately, a lot of what they read here is pure myth.

So before we go any further, I'll take a look at some of these myths and theories, and see what the reality is.

In no particular order, we have:

Fresh fruit & veg is healthier than frozen
Wrong - fresh fruit and vegetables are usually *less* healthy. This is due to a process known as respiration, whereby all fruits and vegetables continue to breathe after being harvested. This breaks down their fat, carbohydrate and protein content, which leads to loss of both flavour and nutrients. It also causes their sugar levels to go up.

However, when they are frozen, the respiration stops, and the sugar and nutrients are preserved at the existing level - sugar low, nutrients high.

Gluten-free diets are healthier
No, they're not. Assuming you don't have an intolerance to gluten, or have Coeliac disease, there is absolutely no reason to remove gluten from your diet. Gluten is found in wheat, barley and rye, which means it's in many carb-based foods, such as biscuits, pies, cakes and pastries. These are all foods you shouldn't be eating, as we'll see later, but the presence of gluten is not the reason.

Saturated fat is bad for you
Most health authorities are still making this claim with regard to heart disease. However, recent studies have demonstrated that it's not true at all. In fact, not only is saturated fat actually good for you, it is absolutely essential. Consider this simple fact - human breast milk is 54 percent saturated fat. Would nature give babies saturated fat if it was bad for them? It is only bad when eaten in excessive quantities - something that applies to all foods!

The studies show that it's actually the trans fats made from vegetable oils, excessive carbohydrate intake, obesity, high blood pressure and sedentary lifestyles that are really behind the heart disease epidemic.

Egg yolks should be avoided
Eggs have been castigated for years because of the high level of cholesterol and saturated fat in the yolks. However, what the health agencies who propagate this nonsense don't tell you, or perhaps aren't even aware of, is that cholesterol is extremely beneficial to your health.

So much so, in fact, the liver actually makes it as very few people get enough through their diet. The more cholesterol you eat, the less has to be made by the liver, and vice versa. In other words, the body always keeps its cholesterol level in balance.

A very large recent study found no association between egg consumption and heart disease or stroke. Other, earlier, studies have reached the same conclusion. Quite clearly, the cholesterol and saturated fat content of eggs isn't an issue.

Carbohydrates are bad for you
This myth has been around for a while now, and is due to the popularity of low-carb diets such as the Atkins. The 'carbs are bad' theory from Dr Atkins and co has led to many people being confused about this foodstuff and its role in our health.

The answer is yes and no. It all depends on the type, quality and amount of carbohydrate being eaten. Carbohydrates that are highly processed, such as those used in biscuits, cereals, breads, cakes, pasta, crackers and so on, have had most, if not all, of the nutrients refined out of them. These foods also have a very high sugar content, which is bad for people as it makes them put on excessive amounts of weight, with the all attendant health issues this brings.

The carbohydrates that *are* good for you are the ones that have either not been processed at all, or just minimally. These do contain nutrients and include all vegetables, fruit, nuts, seeds and legumes.

Salt is bad for you

Not only is salt supposed to be bad for you in general, it can also contribute to cardiovascular disease apparently. However, years of scientific research has failed to show any evidence of this.

Salt is actually an essential nutrient - we simply cannot live without it. A diet too low in salt can give rise to a dangerous condition known as hyponatremia - when the level of sodium in the blood is abnormally low.

Essentially, there are two types of salt - natural salt as found in lakes and the seas, and table salt - highly processed and so far less healthy.

The latter is created by super-heating natural salt, the act of which destroys virtually all its nutrients. The salt is then bleached and cleaned with a chemical solution to make it pure white. Lastly, compounds such as moisture absorbents and anti-caking agents are added to make it easy to pour and sprinkle on food.

While table salt won't give you a stroke or heart attack, neither does it do you any good due to its lack of nutrients. Natural salt, however, does.

A calorie is a calorie is a calorie
It's not, far from it actually. The body stores and utilises calories in various ways that are dependant on the nutrients in the food. As an example, lets compare eating oats and eating fish. Oats contain a type of starch known as 'resistant starch', which is resistant to digestion. Fish, however, doesn't. As a result, the body is unable to absorb and use as many calories from the oats as it can from the fish.

It's a similar story with high-protein foods like poultry. Protein is a high-thermogenic food, which requires an expenditure of energy to digest, absorb and transport it's nutrients to the body's cells. Fats and carbohydrates, on the other hand, are lowthermogenic foods that don't require energy to be used.

Everything else being equal then, calories from fats and carbohydrates will make you gain more weight than an equivalent amount of calories from protein.

Brown bread is better for you than white bread
Indeed it is, assuming you can find some that is actually made with whole grain. Unfortunately, the vast majority of brown bread sold is simply white bread coloured with caramel or molasses to give the appearance of a brown loaf. Nutritionally, it will be no better.

To ensure you don't fall for this con, check the loaf's packaging for the words 'whole grain' or '100% whole wheat'. Also, the first ingredient listed should be a grain of some type, i.e. oats wheat, rye, barley, etc. If it is, you have the genuine article and it will indeed be healthier.

Dairy produce is unhealthy
Another myth perpetuated by the 'saturated fat is bad for you' brigade. Dairy products such as cheese and butter do contain high levels of saturated fat but, as we have already seen, it has now been established that saturated fats are actually very good for us.

Their fat content apart, dairy products are also full of essential nutrients, such as protein, zinc, B vitamins and calcium. Furthermore, weight-loss diets that include dairy produce have been shown to be more effective than diets that omit them.

Organic produce is more nutritious
This one is true but only to a degree. The fact is, the nutritional difference between organically grown and conventionally grown produce is not that great. For most people, it is not enough to justify the expense of going organic. However, for people who take their health seriously, it is, although maybe only just.

It also has to be said that organic food is much less likely to be polluted with pesticides, and so may be worth the extra expense for this reason alone.

You need to drink eight glasses of water a day
Eight glasses is approximately two litres and, together with your water intake from the food you eat and other liquids, is far more than the average person needs. When you need water, your body will tell you - you will suddenly be thirsty - it's as simple as that.

This is a myth propagated by the bottled water industry. When you read this claim, you're reading a marketing stratagem - take no notice.

Eating at night will make you put on weight

Eating at night has long been associated with weight gain. However, the fact is, a calorie is a calorie, regardless of when you eat it. What does make you put on weight is eating more calories than you burn.

It doesn't matter what time of day you eat. It is what and how much you eat, and how much physical activity you do during the day, that determines whether you gain, lose or maintain weight.

Red wine is good for you

There is no question about this - red wine is indeed good for you as it has a high content of antioxidants, such as resveratrol. These fight free radicals (rogue cells that can cause enormous damage) and so reduce the risk of conditions like cancer and heart disease. What's not to like then?

Well, maybe the fact that red wine is, like all alcohol, actually a neurotoxin - a po ison. It may be that the benefits of drinking small amounts (one small glass daily is the suggested limit) outweigh the poisonous effects on the brain. On the other hand, they may not.

As these benefits can also be had by simply eating less and exercising more, why take the risk? If the thought of not drinking alcohol at all bothers you, remember why you're reading this book!

Eat many small meals throughout the day
The theory behind this claim is that by eating more frequently than normal but eating less when you do, your metabolism will remain high. This stops you getting hungry, and also controls your blood sugar level. As a result, you eat less overall and so lose weight.

It's a nice theory but unfortunately it doesn't work in practice. It may raise your metabolism slightly but it's the amount of food eaten that controls hunger levels, not the number of meals.

In fact, research has shown that eating many small meals a day actually makes
people want to eat more - not less.

It should also be pointed out that it's unnatural for our bodies to be constantly in the fed state. In years gone by, it was the norm to go without food for long periods of time, i.e. fast. Research has shown that this is actually good for us.

Low-fat foods are good for you
For a long time now, the mantra has been that people concerned about their weight, or eating for a healthy heart, should eat low-fat foods. As a result, sales of high-fat foods, such as dairy produce, have dropped.

In response, the manufacturers have removed much of the saturated fat from their products in an attempt to make them appear healthier. However, they have replaced the saturated fat with hydrogenated oil (trans fats).

Furthermore, in order to make the low-fat food palatable (most of a food's flavour is in the fat), they have also had to add large amounts of sugar.

What's happened then, is that in these low-fat foods, healthy saturated fats have been replaced with trans fats, refined carbohydrates and sugar - all of which are bad for us. So, they can in fact be positively dangerous.

Omega-6 is bad for you
Omega-6 is a polyunsaturated fat - one of a number of fatty acids found in certain foods, and virtually all vegetable oils.

As to whether it is bad for you, the answer is both yes and no. Omega-6 actually provides many benefits - these include keeping blood pressure low, lowering the risk of heart disease, fighting inflammation, stimulating skin and hair growth, maintaining bone health and many others.

It is, in fact, essential for good health.

The problems come when it is taken in excess, as it is in most western countries, due to it's prevalence in processed foods. All of a sudden, a fat that can be really good for us becomes the instigator of a number of health problems.

These include heart disease, cancer, alzheimer's, rheumatoid arthritis, diabetes and many more.

The polyunsaturated fat most people should be eating a lot more of is omega-3. The ideal ratio of omega-3 to omega-6 fats is 1:1, but in the typical western diet it is between 1:20 and 1:50.

Vegetarian diets are heathier
A vegetarian (vegan) diet consists of nothing but plants, and foods made from plants. Vegans don't eat anything that comes from animals.

The problem with this is that human beings are omnivores - we are designed to function at our best when eating plants *and* animals.

A lot of important nutrients are omitted in a vegetarian diet. Vitamin
B12 is one example - others are protein, vitamin D, iron, zinc and calcium.

There are no studies that show a vegan diet to be healthier than diets that include meat. If a person on a vegan diet is healthy, it's more likely to be because they are health-conscious generally, i.e. they exercise, don't smoke or drink, etc. Not eating meat is immaterial.

The lack of animal nutrients, vitamin B12 and protein in particular, actually makes the vegan diet less healthy. In fact, it can be positively dangerous for children.

All sugar should be avoided
Another word for sugar is energy. And as we all need energy to function, it follows that it can't be bad for us. And indeed, in small amounts, it isn't. Sugar is only a problem when we eat too much of it - as most of us do!

This is because our livers can only deal with a small amount, currently thought to be about six teaspoons a day. Any more is converted into fat.

The problem is exacerbated when we eat refined sugar, such as table sugar. With nothing to slow its absorption, the liver
can be overwhelmed.

When you eat sugar in its natural form - in a piece of fruit for example - you are also eating fibre, minerals and vitamins - these reduce the rate at which the sugar is absorbed in the body, and ease the load on the liver. Plus, the fibre is satiating and so stops you eating too much of the fruit and, hence, sugar.

So remember, as long as you restrict your intake to no more than six teaspoons daily, eating sugar - either natural or refined - won't cause you any problems.